Before you sit down to

to really understand what you are getting yourself
into. This is a life changing process. You will learn
a lot about who you are and who you want to be.
You may see a shift in your priorities. You may see
some things are not really priorities. My goal is
not to change the world. My goal is to help you
find out who you are.

"When you realize nothing is lacking, the whole
world belongs to you." ~Lao Tzu

Mindfulness for beginners:

32 Easy Mindfulness Exercises for Beginners on How to Live Life in the Present Moment, Relieve Stress and Reduce Anxiety.

By

Beatrice Anahata

Table of Contents

How to Fight Cravings with Mindfulness

Basic Techniques To Customize

Just A Final Recap

Some things to think about

mind·ful·ness

ˈmīn(d)f(ə)lnəs/

noun

1.

the quality or state of being conscious or aware of something.

"their mindfulness of the wider cinematic tradition"

2.

a mental state achieved by focusing one's awareness on the present moment, while calmly acknowledging and accepting one's feelings, thoughts, and bodily sensations, used as a therapeutic technique.

Introduction

Getting Started

Life is busy. We have a million things on our to do list, plus another list that doesn't seem to make it to the to do list. Whether you have children, a partner, a full-time job, or it just feels like your life has seemed to slip away from you, meditation can help. Life is overwhelming. It's easy to lose focus. Your mind gets cloudy. Before you know it, it seems like you are just drifting. So now let's get our footing back.

I have to tell you about your room. Right now, it is blank. There isn't anything in there. For the first couple of times, you will need to count to 100 to reach the state of mind that is considered your room. It will be bland. It will be without much to look out, missing colors, and even decorations. Each time that you go, I will point out other things for you to look at and see. Eventually, you will be able to fill in the blanks. Your staircase will change. It may be shorter. There may be a hand rail. Colors will change. Your door may change. You may get to that state of mind one day and you have a pet. You may get there one day and the colors are bright and welcoming. It is your subconscious. It is all about who you are. Let it be. I will say that a lot. Let it be. Why? Because it isn't worth changing. Sometimes you just have to take things as they come. So your two year old wants to wear snow boots in 100 degree weather. Let it be. Just carry shoes with you for when they peel them off. Focus on what you can change. Focus on what you want to change. Only then can you truly be mindful.

The first thing you have to learn is who you are. You need to know what your fears are. You have to know where you are losing your confidence. This first exercise is about self-awakening. I want you to take the time to really focus. Find you a quiet spot. Don't lie down. You will likely fall asleep. Be inspired. If you can't write it out, draw it out. If you do fall asleep, write down your dream as soon as you wake up.

There is no such thing as a failed attempt to mindfulness – just a lack of practice.

<u>Exercise # 1: Facing Who You are</u>

Close your eyes. Take a deep breath. In through your nose and out through your mouth. Imagine in front of your there is a set of stairs. At the top of the stairs in a door. Picture that door. What does it look like? Focus on it as you climb the stairs. Each step you take count. When you get to 100 you should be at the top of the stairs. Welcome to your room. This is your room. Everything about it is your creation. This room holds your happiness, your fears, and even your sadness. There is no stress. There is no judgment. This is all about you. In your room there are three very important things. One is a desk. This is where you will sit and write. You can process everything and nothing just by sitting here. As you focus on your desk, your room will come alive before you. You will notice things about you that you hadn't noticed before. Your desk has drawers. The things stored there are feelings and memories that you have had and haven't wanted to let go off. These control your daily life. You have an unlimited supply of paper and all your favorite writing tools. As you write you will discover the things that you hadn't wanted to face. It's not scary. There is no one here to judge you. It's time to face those fears. Write them. Focus on what you are hiding from yourself. You are in control here. When you are done writing, get up and go to the door. Take each step slowly as you count down from 100.

So, what was this? This was you facing things you didn't want to face. You should have learned more about who you are. Maybe the stress of that day you yelled at your child has been weighing on your heart. Maybe you aren't sure if you are making the right career path. I suggest that you take the time to write this all down. It is definitely going to come pouring out. Release those fears on to your notebook paper. Let them shine. Realize them for what they are or you will never be able to get away from them. It is time for you to be mindful of what you fear so that you can change them.

Exercise #2: The quick trip tip

Let me explain that this is something that you have to do every day but you really need to do it at least once a week or so. It takes ten minutes tops. You can do it quicker or you can take longer but average it to ten minutes.

Close your eyes. Count to ten. Clear your mind completely and totally. Now. Open them and write. Write everything that crosses your mind. Don't think. Don't worry. Definitely don't organize. Just write it all down. When you are finished. Read it. Think about it. Is what you wrote things you can change? Are they things that you want to change? Are they really worth stressing and worrying yourself over?

You need to learn that there will always be things that you will worry about that you just can't change. These are things that, through meditation, you will learn to let go. This is a learning process. You will have to constantly make readjustments to your thinking. That's why it is called the train of thought, because it will stay on the right track, but once you switch the direction, it can be impossible to get back on the right track to your destination. Don't give up, just readjust.

I don't know about you, but for the longest time when I thought of people meditating, I thought about some barely dressed person sitting on a towel with their legs entwined and their fingers touching. It was completely and totally intimidating. I thought, ummm no. I am slightly overweight. I am short. I don't think I want to be half naked on the floor. I will look like a blob. Not to mention, I just am not that religious, so it has to be a complete waste of time. BUTTTTTTT let me tell you something, just please never tell anyone: I WAS WRONG. Yep. Me. I don't admit it often.

What was I wrong about?

1. You don't need to be half naked to find yourself – duh.

2. You don't need to assume any certain position.

3. You don't have to sit on the floor.

4. You don't even need a towel.

5. YOU DO NOT HAVE TO BE LOOKING FOR GOD.

Don't get me wrong. You will find meditation in just about any and every religion. Christian bibles tell you to meditate on the Word of God so that you can engrain them in your heart. Buddhism will tell you to that meditation will lead you to a road of enlightenment. So, what does this teach us? That 1) if you really want something to be a part of you, meditate on it 2) that if you meditate, you will find your path.

Speaking of path, that brings me to:

<u>Exercise #3: The path</u>

Here I am not talking about what person to date. I am talking about life changing decisions that will ultimately guide you to where you need to be. It's like choosing between that job in California and the one in New York. It is the twisting turning, they both have good sides, path.

Count to ten. Take deep steady breaths. Imagine in front of you are the woods. With each and every step, you are deeper in the woods. At ten, STOP. Look around. You see two paths you can take. One path looks bright and sunny. The other path looks shady and cool. Pick on and take a walk down it. Keep your mind clear. Just focus on your steps. The smells of the woods are around you. Enjoy your journey. Each step brings you closer to your destiny. When you get to the end of your path, what do you see? Write it down. Which one of your choices does it resemble the most?

Exercise #4: Imagining your life

Take a minute. Focus on what you love about your life right now. Think about all the things you never want to change. What do you love about your house? Your routine? Now think about one of your options. How will those things change? How will that become better? What will come worse? Now, thing about your other choice. Ask yourself the same questions. Do you see the clear difference?

I always tend to go to the method 4 when I am really wanting a change for the better. I always get stuck in a routine that gets boring. On the other hand, change can be downright terrifying. These steps help to take the guesswork out of it and help to solidify what I need to do so that I can do it with no issues. A little peace of mind goes a long way.

The Situation of It All

Here is the crazy thing about life. It is always the most stressful in short bursts that make you wonder if you are going to lose your mind before you manage to get through it. These short bursts sometimes only last minutes or hours. By the end of the day, or maybe the week, everything comes into perspective and you realize it wasn't so bad after all. So now I will take the time to go over some situations that seem so very bad and show you how to be **MINDFUL** of your temporary situation so that you make it through without falling apart.

So here you are at the grocery store. You really only wanted to pick up a few things and be on your way. So you make your way to the register and there is that woman there. You know which one I am talking about. The one with two basket full of groceries. She has a one screaming kid and one kid going through the candy like it has never eaten before. It is the only register open. Then just when you think it's almost over, she pulls out her coupon book. The manager gets called over to take her complaint and you really want to just scream. However you could just use:

Exercise #5:

Take a deep breath. Slowly count. If the kid hears you, they will probably get out of the candy, but don't focus on that. Just count your breaths. Think to yourself, be peaceable with all mankind. In and out. You will feel your mind clear. You will see the light at the end of the tunnel. Just like that and your aisle is clear. See, that wasn't so bad, now was it?

Sitting at your desk at work. Your desk is piled up with a million papers for you to look at. You have an inbox that will take you until lunch to get through. There is a meeting after lunch. You have no idea how you are going to get it all done. So how about:

Exercise #6:

Stop what you are doing and breath. Picture yourself in an empty field. Imagine the wind blowing. Count up to 100. Say to yourself: I am at peace. This is no big deal. Feel the tension relax out of your body. Clear mind. Clear body. Keep counting until you find all your stress just go away.

It has been a long day. The kids are running around everywhere. You just want to stop and relax. It seems like the more stressful day you have a work, the more there is to do at home. It never stops. However:

Exercise #7:

can help you to reset your mind. All you have to do is stop. Sit down. Calmly begin to count. You can count out loud if you would like. Your kids may need a quick reset. So just count. Breath steady and clearly. Stop counting when you feel your mind reset and your body relax. You are now ready to continue.

You are late. You forgot to set your alarm, or maybe you turned it off in your sleep. Either way, you are definitely not going to make it to your shift on time. And now you are stuck in traffic. As far as you can see there is nothing but tail lights. So you could scream – it won't do any good. Or you could do:

Exercise #8:

Turn on some classical music. It is always calming. Don't close your eyes. It would be not so smart while you are driving. Just focus your energy on relaxing. Count to 100. Take steady, even breaths. Focus on releasing the stress out of your soul. Feel your mind clearing. Feel you mind preparing for a positive day.

You are balancing your checking account. You definitely don't see how you are going to make it. The stress of the bills are weighing you down. You can try:

Exercise #9:

Think about what you want to accomplish. Visualize it and focus on it. Imagine your bank account balancing. Clear your mind. Feel the stress melt away. You will see that it will all come together. A plan will form and your stress will go away.

Social anxiety sucks. It is so hard to deal with. You want to go out. You want people to like you, but you just can't get past the inability to breathe. Your palms get sweaty. You feel like you don't make any sense. Overall, you are just plain awkward. You have gone over all the conversation starters you can possibly think of, but nothing sounds natural. So it is time for:

Exercise #10:

Take a deep breath. Listen to your heart. Know who you are. Think of all the great things you have to offer to the conversation. Count back from 20 and feel the anxiety roll away. Before you know it, you are a new person. You are ready for the conversation. Jump in and don't be afraid of the silence from time to time.

It is time to cram for that test. You are on your third pot of coffee and none of the information is sticking. Your eyes just want to close. Don't give up yet. I know a technique that may help you. I had a friend that swore he could write things on his chalkboard and never forget them. So here is:

Exercise #11:

Close your eyes. Take a deep breath. In through your nose and out through your mouth. Imagine in front of your there is a set of stairs. At the top of the stairs in a door. Picture that door. What does it look like? Focus on it as you climb the stairs. Each step you take count. When you get to 100 you should be at the top of the stairs. Welcome to your room. This is your room. Everything about it is your creation. This room holds your happiness, your fears, and even your sadness. There is no stress. There is no judgment.

This is all about you. In your room there are three very important things. One is a desk. You already know about the desk so we are going to ignore it for now. Look at your walls. There is a chalkboard on one of them. Visualize yourself writing on this chalkboard. Picture each and every word as you write it. This will ingrain it into your memory. Write down all the important things that you know you will need for your exam. Make charts. Keep it simple. You will see that it will all come together. When you are finished, you will feel more confident and prepared for your exam.

While you are in your room, look at the bookcase behind you. It is massive. It takes up the entire wall. On it is every book you ever wrote. Each book is a year of your life. Some of the books are thick, they contain life experiences. They lay out exactly what you think you learned from that experience. Take the time to look them over. You may find that you overlooked a lesson. Now, count back from 100 and return to your life. Feel refreshed and ready to face the world.

I would love to tell you all about my room. I would love to tell you the details. The colors that come to life when I visit it. I cannot. I do not want to influence your room. I want you to create it yourself. So, please enjoy it.

Meditation is amazing. It is an amazing tool. I hope that you can use these to get through some common stresses at the very moment that you are going through them. I think that it would help you to better understand that you are dealing with temporary problems. Your life can change dramatically from one minute to the next. Next year will be completely different, so don't focus on anything other than right now. Make each and every moment stress free. You are the only one that can do this. Only you can control what worries you. My mom always told me, don't stress over the apple pie burning when you know you are going to be enjoying the smell of it all through the house. It means, why worry about something when you know you are doing the best that you can to make sure that it never turns out that way.

Life is hard enough without stressing over every detail.

The Seven Forms Of Meditation: Quick Guide

Transcendental Meditation – Exercise #12

You will see this among the traditional Hindu. So this is basically chanting your way over the stress. You repeat the same mantra over and over again until you achieve a higher state of mind. You want to place the negative aspects at the bottom and rise above it. The easiest way to do this is to download a video. You can do it as a beginner, but it isn't as easy. I highly suggest this if you are a hands on type of learner because you have to focus your mind to repeat the words exactly so that they begin to consume you completely. It is a thing of beauty once you master it. It does take lots of practice. You should start of doing this out loud, which is fine in the car, but will get you some strange looks at work. Your kids probably wouldn't notice or think you are losing your mind, but that's okay.

Heart Rhythm Meditation – Exercise #13

I don't suggest this to beginners. It is the focus of the heart rhythm in order to guide you to a higher state of mind. You have to really focus on your heart and allow your breathing to sync with it. It can be quite difficult to achieve, but if you do, it is the ultimate in soul awakening experiences. You will find that you are happier when you learn to do it regularly. It is a whole body experience.

Kundalini – Exercise #14

is just a little bit different than all the rest. It is really simple. All you really need to do is focus on the very center of your body. Concentrate until you find the core of your breathing. Feel your stress uncoiling from there and floating to the outside of your body. You want to literally feel your stress rising up out of the center of your body and leaving you completely and totally. You will feel lighter. You will feel more free. You may even find who you are.

Guided Visualization – Exercise #15

This may not be what you are looking for if you are reading this book. Let me tell you why. You have to have the visual. You need to be walked through each and every step. Listen to a recording of yourself being guided through visualizing your problems away. It is time consuming. I don't like it. I don't even know if I like it being number 16. The reason it is listed is because it is real. It can help you, but you cannot do it on your own. It isn't a quick fix. It will lead you to self awareness, destress you, and make you happy. Just make sure you get a voice that you like to hear the sound of, or record yourself and listen to it later. That would make it easier for you, maybe. I just know that this one is not for me.

Qi Gong – Exercise #16

This exercise comes from the Chinese idea that all your body systems are connected. It is called the whole body approach to health. It is directed at releasing negative energy so that your body can heal itself. A stressed body is a sick body. Your focus needs to be on breathing techniques. You want to breath and direct energy to each part of your body. It will sync your healing so that your stress is released and your mind is clear which will allow your energy to focus on healing your body. It is so simple. You just deep breath and focus on your aches and relax them. Your body will feel energized.

Zazen – Exercise #17

This is the Zen method borrowed from Buddha. You are supposed to sit in the legs crossed position in the floor to keep your energy flowing in the circle of your body. You want to sit with your legs crossed and your hands in your lap. You need to focus all your thoughts into releasing the negative ideas, comments, and thoughts from your head completely. You should focus on breathing until you feel released and free. At first, it may be difficult to achieve that perfect peace quickly, but as you practice, you will get there quicker and quicker.

Traditional Western – Exercise #18

The thing is that this is where mindfulness comes from. It is simple. It is teaching your mind to refocus off the negativity and refocus on its ability to find the good in the situation. It encompasses all forms of meditation. It is the simple calming of your spirit to enjoy who you are. Simple deep breathing to readjust your train of thought. It is taking five minutes to reorganize your priorities. It is loving yourself. Just breath until you feel settled.

How to Fight Cravings with Mindfulness

Fight Cravings – Exercise #19

No matter what you are trying to do, or not do, mindfulness can help. You can calm your craving for a cigarette. You can break your addiction to food. There are many ways to use The very second that you feel your craving coming on, focus on it. Feel the craving in your body. Feel the tingle. Feel the ability to fight it. It is real. It is a chemical part of your body. Now focus on it. Make up your mind that your ultimate outcome is far more beneficial than giving into this single craving. Allow it to dissolve. Release it from your body. You will begin to notice that space between cravings is getting bigger. Soon they will be gone altogether. You can do this.

Awaken Your Senses – Exercise #20

Are you feeling bad? Do you feel sluggish and want a new outlook? Let's try to awaken your senses. You may be surprised at how much better you can feel from this simple I want you to find somewhere quiet. Light a candle. Now. Let's start with your sense of smell. I want you to think about exactly how that candle smells. What are the other scents in the room? Can you smell anything outside of the room? Taste. Can you taste the scent of the candle? What does it remind you of? Touch. Can you feel the heat off the candle? Does it add to the taste? Does it take away from the taste? Hear. What sounds can you hear that the candle makes you think of? How does it tie in with the taste, touch, and smell of the room around you? Finally, what can you see in your mind's eye that brings everything home? What has this experience taught you about who you are? What has it taught you about the world around you? How can you use this in your mindful meditation later? This is all about reopening your senses because we tend to shut them down and get tunnel vision.

Sleep Better – Exercise #21

Now let's use mindfulness to help you to fight your insomnia and stay asleep so that your body can reach REM state. Without that precious REM state, your body cannot rejuvenate. Lay down. Focus on your breathing. Concentrate on how your abdomen muscles expand with each breath. Imagine your breath coming out your mouth. In with your nose. Steady pattern. Regular breathing is a must. Now focus on your toes. Wiggle them slightly. Release the tension in them. Move up your legs. Release the stress in them. Move through your body. Focus on each part. Release the stress from each pocket. Find the stress points and gently massage them with your mind. If your mind begins to wander to current events in your life, gently refocus it and bring it back to where it was. It is all about relaxing and letting the day go. Every time that you exhale, release the stress out with the bad air. You can do this every night. Soon your body will be trained to let everything go as soon as you lay in bed at night. Your sleepless nights are soon to be a thing of the past. Remember to try to keep a dream journal when you wake up in the morning. Dreams are just your subconscious trying to tell you something or release the drama in your life. You would be surprised at the power of your dreams in your daily life. Keeping track of them will help you to find your way if you are feeling lost or confused – but that is for another book at another time.

Controlling Your Thoughts and Emotions – Exercise #22

I know that this is the hardest part of life. It isn't easy to control your judgment of your own thoughts. I know that sounds weird, but we are our biggest enemy. We hold ourselves back. is all about thinking about what your mind wants to think about. Just letting thoughts flow. Sit in a way that you will feel comfortable.

Focus on just breathing, such as the feeling of the air flowing into your nose and out through your mouth. Once you have focused your concentration fully. Focus on your thoughts. Become aware of sounds, sensations, and ideas within your own head.

Let each thought flow without deciding if it is good or bad. If your thoughts flow to fast refocus your breathing. Then begin all over again.

Let me think. We covered common stressful situations. We have covered tricks to help common problems. I have compartmentalized the absolute best that I could. So I guess now I can just give you the techniques. These are basics that can cover anything. They can be completely personalized. They can handle whatever you want. They are the basics.

Basic Techniques To Customize

Deep Breathing – Exercise #23

Deep breathing is taking slow, deep, methodical mouthfuls of air and slow exhalations. You can do it for as you want to. If your mind wanders simply try to refocus on your breathing.

- ☯ Inhale through your nose.

- ☯ Feel your breath travel down into your stomach. Feel your lungs expand.

- ☯ Focus on the ambiences of breathing deeply and slowly.

- ☯ You will be able to feel your body rise and fall on each draw of your breath.

- ☯

Doing a Seated Meditation – Exercise #24

Find a quiet spot. You can meditate anywhere. However, you will probably want to be somewhere you won't be distracted. You want somewhere comfortable. Even if that is just closing the door to your office. You could just take a walk to a nearby park or library.

- ☯ Turn off all your electronics just to keep them from bothering.

- ☯ Give yourself 5 or ten minutes. Get comfortable. You just need a position that will help you to relax.

- ☯ When you're comfortable close your eyes.

- ☯ Focus on your breath. Block out any other thoughts. Any time you find your mind wandering, simply return your focus.

- ☯ Take deep breaths that go all the way down to your abdomen.

- Feel the air flow through your nostrils and into your lungs.

- Notice the feeling of your chest rising and falling with each inhalation and exhalation.

- You can set a timer for 5 to 10 minutes, but I prefer to breathe until I feel a sense of peace come over me.

- You can take these little meditation breaks anytime you want to.

- Open your eyes. When you're finished, slowly open your eyes. Don't get up right away. Just give your mind time to readjust to the peace.

- Stand up slowly.

Visualization Meditation – Exercise # 25

Get relaxed and breathe intensely. Use deep breathing exercises, just like you have already learned in the rest of the book.

Sit in a quiet spot and remove as many distractions as you can. Turn off your cellphone and find somewhere you can be alone just for a few minutes.

- Release any tight clothing.

- You can visualize whatever you want. It can be a real place you have been, or your own imaginary world. Really focus so that your mind thinks it is there.

- Start by picturing a visual image in your head. Choose a place that is totally relaxing. Think of all the things that you imagine would make the place peaceful.

- Imagine the sounds you'd hear there.

- Next, imagine the physical sensations you might experience there.

- Open your eyes and stand up slowly.

Mindful Observation – Exercise #26

This exercise is unassuming but unbelievably influential. It is designed to all us to connect us with the natural environment, which is so easy for us to forget to do on a regular basis.

Choose an ordinary object from your direct atmosphere and focus on watching it. This could be a living thing like a flower or your child or even just the clouds in the sky.

Don't do anything else. Focus on only the thing you are looking at. Simply relax into a peaceful state for as long as you possibly can. Look at it as if you have never seen it before.. Visually explore every part of its being. Let it take over your mind completely and totally. Connect with its energy and purpose in your world.

Mindful Awareness – Exercise #27

Think of something that you do every day, more than once a day. Or focus on something that happens several times throughout the day. It should be something that you sometimes forget to notice or take for granted that will always be there. Like maybe the refrigerator light.

Think about how much harder life would be without it. Or doorknobs, what would you do without them? What would a door look like? It makes you really appreciate the little things in life. Change it every day. Like maybe the smell of you cooking can remind you to be thankful that you have food to cook or children to feed. Or when you notice your spouse forgot to get gas, redirect that thought and be thankful you have the vehicle that needs gas.

Mindful Listening – Exercise #28

Pick a song that you have never heard before. It could be on the radio or maybe just something on your playlist that you haven't listened to yet. Close your eyes. Put in your ear-buds. Listen to the song. Even if you don't really like it at first, just listen. All your soul to reach down into the song and feel the beat. Let it consume your mind until you feel like you are one with the music.

Mindful Immersion – Exercise #29

Through yourself into a task. It doesn't matter what it is. Just give yourself over to it completely. If it is cleaning the floor, then just focus on appreciating the way that it looks clean. Appreciate the way that the sun shines on it. Appreciate the colors in it. The beauty of it. If you do this then your daily routines won't seem so routine any more.

Mindful Appreciation #30

Find five things that you are thankful for. I do it every night before I go to bed. It really helps to melt away the stress and the headaches. You could stop every time you are frustrated and find five reason why you love your life. You can look around your messy house and find five reasons why you love the mess. You can look at your spouse who won't decide what to have for dinner and just start telling them the five reasons that you love them. It is all about refocusing on who you are and why you love your life. It is about living in the moment.

Mindful brushing —Exercise #31

Sometimes we just get caught up in the routine of it all. We move through the motions, like when we brush or teeth or hair. Our mind will wonder and we will start to think about our worries, regrets, hopes, and fears. But what if you could take that time and refocus it in to a happy place? I want you to just focus on the art of brushing your teeth. Notice how it feels. Notice how it tastes. Really focus on that experience. It is a human experience. It is one we take for granted.

The Eating Exercise – Exercise #32

This is to bring your mind to what is right in front of you. You can pick any food you want. It is just a focus item. I want you to notice how it looks. Take in every single bump, curve, texture. Notice how it really feels, smooth, rough, and everything in between. How does it move when you touch it. Notice how the skin gives a little. Or how it doesn't give at all. Notice the smell. Then the taste. Focus on it totally and completely.

Just A Final Recap

I want to remind you that this is a journey that is all about you. It isn't about me. It isn't about your neighbor. It is about rediscovering what you love about your life. Mindfulness can help in so many ways.

It can

- Help you to de-stress

- Help you to realize your full potential

- Help you to realize your dreams

- Help you to reach your goals

- Help you to break addictions

- Help you to feel better

It cannot

- Change who you are at your core

- Change the people around you

- Change your situation

- Change your environment

I STRONGLY urge you to try all the techniques until you find one that you love. It is about you being happy. You will absolutely find what you are looking for, if it is within you. You won't get rich, but you may find it easier to manage money. It can't make your boss promote you, but it can give you an attitude change that may help you earn that promotion. It is about finding yourself. So please take time to focus on yourself. Love yourself first.

Some things to think about

I am including some quotes because sometimes you need something inspiring to really think about. I hope that you find one that really speaks to you and can help your center when everything else is falling apart. My favorite quote came from a TV show " Saved by the Bell" when I was 11 years old. I still tell myself this every single time I think about giving up. Now, I will tell you my trials have deepened over the years but this one quote has grown with me and changed meanings many times throughout the years. "Put your mind to it, go for, get down and break a sweat. Rock and Roll, You ain't seen nothing yet"

Here are some classics:

- ☯ Drink your tea slowly and reverently, as if it is the axis on which the world earth revolves – slowly, evenly, without rushing toward the future; live the actual moment. Only this moment is life." ~Thich Nhat Hanh."

- "As soon as we wish to be happier, we are no longer happy." ~Walter Landor

- "Mindfulness is the aware, balanced acceptance of the present experience. It isn't more complicated than that. It is opening to or receiving the present moment, pleasant or unpleasant, just as it is, without either clinging to it or rejecting it." ~Sylvia Boorstein

- "The best way to capture moments is to pay attention. This is how we cultivate mindfulness. Mindfulness means being awake. It means knowing what you are doing." ~Jon Kabat-Zinn

- "In today's rush, we all think too much — seek too much — want too much — and forget about the joy of just being." ~Eckhart Tolle

- "If you want others to be happy, practice compassion. If you want to be happy, practice compassion." ~Dalai Lama

- "Suffering usually relates to wanting things to be different than they are." ~Allan Lokos

- "If we learn to open our hearts, anyone, including the people who drive us crazy, can be our teacher." ~Pema Chodron

- "If the doors of perception were cleansed, everything would appear to man as it is, infinite." ~William Blake

- "Feelings come and go like clouds in a windy sky. Conscious breathing is my anchor." ~Thich Nhat Han

- "If you want to conquer the anxiety of life, live in the moment, live in the breath." ~Amit Ray

- "In the end, just three things matter: How well we have lived. How well we have

loved. How well we have learned to let go"
~Jack Kornfield

- "Do every act of your life as though it were the last act of your life." ~Marcus Aurelius

- "Everything is created twice, first in the mind and then in reality." ~Robin S. Sharma

- "Don't believe everything you think. Thoughts are just that – thoughts." ~Allan Lokos

- "Respond; don't react. Listen; don't talk. Think; don't assume." ~Raji Lukkoor

- "In this moment, there is plenty of time. In this moment, you are precisely as you should be. In this moment, there is infinite possibility." ~Victoria Moran

- "Mindfulness is simply being aware of what is happening right now without wishing it were different; enjoying the pleasant without holding on when it changes (which it will); being with the unpleasant without fearing it will always be this way (which it won't)." ~James Baraz

- "Mindfulness isn't difficult, we just need to remember to do it." ~Sharon Salzberg

- "It's only when we truly know and understand that we have a limited time on earth – and that we have no way of knowing when our time is up – that we will begin to live each day to the fullest, as if it was the only one we had." ~Elisabeth Kübler-Ross

- "Begin at once to live, and count each separate day as a separate life." ~Seneca

- "Today, like every other day, we wake up empty and frightened. Don't open the door to the study and begin reading. Take down a musical instrument." ~Rumi

☯ "I wish that life should not be cheap, but sacred. I wish the days to be as centuries, loaded, fragrant." ~Ralph Waldo Emerson

☯ "Each morning we are born again. What we do today is what matters most." ~Buddha

☯ "Always hold fast to the present. Every situation,indeed every moment,is of infinite value,for it is the representative of a whole eternity." ~Johann Wolfgang von Goethe

☯ "The way to live in the present is to remember that 'This too shall pass.' When you experience joy, remembering that 'This too shall pass' helps you savor the here and now. When you experience pain and sorrow, remembering that 'This too shall pass' reminds you that grief, like joy, is only temporary." ~Joey Green

☯ "If you concentrate on finding whatever is good in every situation, you will discover that your life will suddenly be filled with gratitude, a feeling that nurtures the soul." ~Rabbi Harold Kushner

- "There's only one reason why you're not experiencing bliss at this present moment, and it's because you're thinking or focusing on what you don't have.... But, right now you have everything you need to be in bliss." ~Anthony de Mello

- "Our own worst enemy cannot harm us as much as our unwise thoughts. No one can help us as much as our own compassionate thoughts." ~Buddha

- "Observe the space between your thoughts, then observe the observer." ~Hamilton Boudreaux

- "The practice of mindfulness begins in the small, remote cave of your unconscious mind and blossoms with the sunlight of your conscious life, reaching far beyond

the people and places you can see."
~Earon Davis

❧ "Life is not lost by dying; life is lost minute by minute, day by dragging day, in all the small uncaring ways." ~Stephen Vincent Benet

❧ "As long as we have practiced neither concentration nor mindfulness, the ego takes itself for granted and remains its usual normal size, as big as the people around one will allow." ~Ayya Khema

❧ "Impermanence is a principle of harmony. When we don't struggle against it, we are in harmony with reality." ~Pema Chodron

❧ The basic root of happiness lies in our minds; outer circumstances are nothing more than adverse or favorable." ~Matthieu Ricard

❧ "The mind in its natural state can be compared to the sky, covered by layers of cloud which hide its true nature." ~Kalu Rinpoche

☯ "Be kind whenever possible. It is always possible." ~Dalai Lama

☯ "If one were truly aware of the value of human life, to waste it blithely on distractions and the pursuit of vulgar ambitions would be the height of confusion." ~Dilgo Khyentse Rinpoche

☯ "Knowledge does not mean mastering a great quantity of different information, but understanding the nature of mind. This knowledge can penetrate each one of our thoughts and illuminate each one of our perceptions." ~Matthieu Ricard

☯ "The most precious gift we can offer others is our presence. When mindfulness embraces those we love, they will bloom like flowers." ~Thich Nhat Hanh

- "We are awakened to the profound realization that the true path to liberation is to let go of everything." ~Jack Kornfield

- "To diminish the suffering of pain, we need to make a crucial distinction between the pain of pain, and the pain we create by our thoughts about the pain. Fear, anger, guilt, loneliness and helplessness are all mental and emotional responses that can intensify pain." ~Howard Cutler

- "Things falling apart is a kind of testing and also a kind of healing." ~Pema Chodron

- "Why, if we are as pragmatic as we claim, don't we begin to ask ourselves seriously: Where does our real future lie?" ~Sogyal Rinpoche

- "Envy and jealousy stem from the fundamental inability to rejoice at

someone else's happiness or success."
~Matthieu Ricard

☯ "By breaking down our sense of self-importance, all we lose is a parasite that has long infected our minds. What we gain in return is freedom, openness of mind, spontaneity, simplicity, altruism: all qualities inherent in happiness."
~Matthieu Ricard

☯ "Our lives are lived in intense and anxious struggle, in a swirl of speed and aggression, in competing, grasping, possessing and achieving, forever burdening ourselves with extraneous activities and preoccupations." ~Sogyal Rinpoche

☯ "Mindful and creative, a child who has neither a past, nor examples to follow, nor value judgments, simply lives, speaks and plays in freedom." ~Arnaud Desjardins

☯ "We have only now, only this single
eternal moment opening and unfolding
before us, day and night." Jack Kornfield